How To Stop Worrying And Start Living:

The Most Effective Permanent Solution To Finally Overcome Worrying And Start Living

Table of Contents

Introduction 5

Chapter 1: Identifying Sources of Worry in Your Life 6

    Identifying Sources of Stress: 6

    Making a List: 6

    Top 3 Stresses: 6

    Some Worry is Healthy: 7

    Reducing Sources of Stress: 7

    Picking a Start Date: 7

Chapter 2: Getting Your Life In Order 9

    Helping Others by Donating: 9

    Volunteer Work: 10

    Reaching Out for Help: 10

    Staying Away from Negative Influences: 11

    Making a Good First Impression: 11

Chapter 3: Tips To Relieve Stress 13

    Focus on Positive Thoughts: 13

    Reduce Stress by Exercising: 13

    Relaxing Music: 14

    Laughter is Good Medicine: 14

    Meditate: 14

    Slow Down: 15

    Staying Connected: 15

    Helping Others: 15

Chapter 4: Finding Balance In Your Life 16
   Positive Relationships with Others: 16
   Get Out of the House: 16
   Well Rested: 17
   Healthy Daily Habits: 17
   Stay Away from Alcohol: 17
   Joining A Support Group: 18
   Balancing Work and Play: 18

Chapter 5: Trying To Eat The Stress Away 19
   Feel Better or Comfort Foods: 19
   Choose a Healthy Snack: 19
   Food the Modifier: 19
   Magnesium Mood Booster: 20
   Omega- 3's Reduce Depression: 20
   Nutritional Balance will Improve Emotional Balance: 20

Chapter 6: Remember To Be Grateful 21
   Think of Others Who are in Need: 21
   Stop Feeling Sorry for Yourself: 22
   Show Compassion Towards Others: 22
   Remember to Tell Your Loved Ones You Love Them: 23
   Giving Thanks Daily: 23

Chapter 7: How Is Worrying Related To Living? 25

Chapter 8: What Are The Primary Causes Of Worry? 29
   Insecurity 29
   Jealousy 30

Competitions 32

Stress and strain 33

Priorities 34

Expectations 35

Survival 36

Chapter 9: How To Minimize Or Eliminate Worry From Your Life? 38

Food 38

Planning 39

Socialization 40

Escape 42

Positivity 42

Learn to say no 44

Develop hobbies 45

Professional life v. Personal life 45

Yoga 46

Stay healthy, if not fit 47

Chapter 10: How To Prevent Worries From Aggravating 49

First stage: Identification 49

Second stage: Treatment 49

Third stage: Alienation 50

Fourth stage: Unconscious imbibing of the three stages 50

Chapter 11: How Would Stopping Worrying Help You With Start Living? 52

Conclusion 57

Introduction

I want to thank you and congratulate you for downloading the book, "How to Stop Worrying and Start Living".

This book contains proven steps and strategies on how to leave behind old habits and behaviors and adopt new ones, better for you.

You can learn how to trade bad habits for good habits just by following some of the positive suggestions given in this book. Change is never usually easy but when it is for the better of your over-all well being then it is well worth the effort.

If you truly want to be able to worry less and enjoy life more then I suggest that you start by reading this book. This book will be a wonderful tool to help guide you to that calm more peaceful way of living; you owe it to yourself to learn to worry less and start living.

Take the first step towards a life you can truly begin to enjoy by reading the steps and strategies this book offers on how to achieve the desired results that you are seeking.

Thanks again for downloading this book, I hope you enjoy it!

Bonus – Buy This Book And Get a Free Report!!

Chapter 1:
Identifying Sources of Worry in Your Life

Identifying Sources of Stress:

The first step towards living a more relaxed and happy life is to try and identify the chief sources of stress in your life. A good idea is to sit down and make a list of the things that cause you great worry and concern. Now, when writing this list, don't add things on it that are not within your control to change such as the weather for example. Try and include things that are within your grasp to change such as your diet. If you are worrying that you may be too overweight and that your health is suffering because of it well this is something you can change.

Making a List:

A good idea when composing your list is to start with a small number of goals and as you progress and conquer one goal you can add a new goal in its place. As the saying goes 'there is always room for improvement'. Perhaps pick the top 3 things in your life that you worry about the most; put them in an order 1-3 one being the most worrisome. Start by trying to find ways to make your no.1 stress a less stressful part of your life.

Top 3 Stresses:

As individuals we all have different areas in our lives that stress us more than others. There are areas that are common stresses in most people's lives three of the top ones being financial, health issues and personal relationships. I believe the majority of us have at one point or another experienced excess worry in one or all of these 3 areas. Having stress in our lives is part of life but we must learn how to manage our stress levels in more positive and productive ways.

Some Worry is Healthy:

To have some worry is healthy as it helps to prepare us for unexpected stressful events in our lives. As we know too much of anything is not good and this includes too much worry. Finding a healthy balance is the key to reaching a more relaxed and calm way of living and being able to enjoy life to the fullest. Teaching yourself to look at things in a more positive light over negative is an important step in the right direction.

How you view the world in general has a great effect on your well being as a whole. If you are always worrying about one thing after the other you are affecting your mental and physical state of being in a negative way. This constant stress on your body can lead to triggering other health issues.

Reducing Sources of Stress:

Once you have decided what causes you the most worry in your life you must then think of things you can do to reduce the sources of this particular worry. Try and decide what you can do to make it a less stressful part of your life. If you are unsure that is okay because this book will give you some great suggestions on things you can do to help lessen your stress in different areas.

Picking a Start Date:

Another good idea is to pick a start date not unlike when someone is going on a diet they quite often will pick a start date. This helps to get you prepared mentally for the challenge ahead. Remember to start small with your challenges and as you progress add more once you feel comfortable enough to do so. Make your goals ones that are realistic for you do not make them too unattainable as you are just setting yourself up for failure.

Remember 'Rome wasn't built in a day' and either will your lifestyle change. It will take a certain level of self discipline and control on your part to succeed at your goals. Starting with small goals will help to build your self-confidence up which will help to give you the courage and stamina to continue moving forward to conquering bigger goals. By reading this book you are taking very important steps that will lead you towards enjoy living life more and worrying less.

Chapter 2:
Getting Your Life In Order

Organize and Clean Home:

A great place to start your journey towards a less worrisome and stress filled life is to start with your home and getting it organized. If you have things piling up within your home most of which you have not used in a year chances are these are things you do not really need or use. Time to do a spring cleaning of sorts; you must be willing to part with items in order to accomplish the goal of getting your house in order.

This can be a great source of stress causing you to worry that you will never be able to organize the disarray within your home. Constantly going through this ritual time and time again is causing you unnecessary stress. You can reduce your stress and worry enormously by getting rid of the excess disorganized clutter within your home. Things that you no longer use you may want to consider donating them. If you are not comfortable with donating them then perhaps you should try to organize a garage sale and sell the excess of things you no longer use.

Helping Others by Donating:

If you have a garage sale and there is stuff left over from the sale you really should consider donating this stuff. Just think that it will be going to people who will make good use of it instead of it gathering dust within your home. You can feel good in knowing you are doing a good deed by donating clothing, furniture etc. to those who are in need.

Helping others who are less fortunate than yourself is a great form of therapy in making yourself feel better that you are doing a good deed. It is a great way to worry less about your own problems when you help others that are much worse off than yourself. You soon realize that the small problems and worries you have are nothing in comparison to what someone who is less fortunate than yourself has to deal on a daily basis.

Volunteer Work:

Doing a volunteer job is a great way to help you through helping others. When you are helping others who are less fortunate than yourself you realize how lucky you are to have the life that you have it may not be perfect but there is many who would trade places with you in a heartbeat.

When doing volunteer work you will be too busy helping others to have time to spend sitting around feeling sorry for yourself or worrying about all that is not right in your own life. By giving your help and time freely to others you are also giving yourself a positive experience that will make you feel good about yourself. You will look at yourself as a person that is helping others instead of a selfish person always worrying and stressing about your own imperfections and missing out on enjoying life.

Reaching Out for Help:

Perhaps you can go to friends and family members and tell them you want to make some positive changes in your life. Explain to them that you want to start by getting your home in order. If you reach out to others and ask for help there is many who would be more than glad to help you in your time of need. Your friends and loved ones would love to see you worrying less and living and loving life more; instead of watching you burying yourself alive in worry and stress.

You could also seek professional help in getting counseling about your over stressing tendencies. If they have really gotten to an extreme level where you have basically cut yourself off from friends and loved ones due to your negative behavior then you should seek some outside help.

If you seek some counseling you can get some great advice from counselors on what the best approach would be for you. Explain to them how you tend to spend more time worrying about things rather than trying to enjoy life. They can help you to stop bad habits and replace them with some good habits.

Staying Away from Negative Influences:

In order for you to make a start you must stay away from any negative influences in your life. If there is people in your life that are always putting you down and making you feel like you cannot accomplish anything worthwhile then these are not your friends. Friends would be trying to give you positive support. You need to surround yourself with positive people that will encourage you to move forward and do better for yourself. People that truly care about you will not want to see you in a worried stressed out state unable to enjoy life. They instead will want to see you enjoying life to the fullest!

Making a Good First Impression:

Getting your home in order it will give you the confidence you need to continue on towards a positive lifestyle. Whether you are interacting with people on a personal level or a business level you should want to make a good impression. You should make sure that your home is organized and clean when inviting people to come into your home because your home is an extension of yourself. How your home is kept is a reflection on how you are viewed by others. People will look at the state your home is in to get a sense of what kind of person you are. You will feel less stress and anxiety when people visit if your house is organized; it doesn't have to be perfect but having some order is better than complete disorder.

Now that you have completed the first stage towards achieving a life of worrying less the next step will give you suggestions on how to meditate and exercise so that you can learn how to relax your mind and body. This will eventually enable you to reach a state of calm and relaxation. Once your home environment is a calm and peaceful place it will be time to move forward to the next phase of your journey of relaxing your mind and body so you will worry less and start living!

Chapter 3:
Tips To Relieve Stress

Time to learn a few great suggestions in obtaining a calm and relaxed state; just remember these tips are good for you and don't take long to do. You can achieve a certain level of relaxation within 15 minutes. So why not treat yourself and try some of these wonderful stress relievers.

Focus on Positive Thoughts:

Try to think of the things that you are grateful for in your life, count your blessings and any negative thoughts or worries push them aside. Keeping a journal(s) can help you to remind yourself of all the blessings in your life by writing them down, also add in your journal any positive accomplishments you have made and celebrate them. At times when you are feeling really worried or stressed look through your journals notes to remind yourself of things that truly matter in your life.

Reduce Stress by Exercising:

Many forms of exercising are great to help in the lowering of anxiety as well as depression because during this time the brain releases chemicals that make us feel good. This feel good feeling we get while exercising is known as a runner's high. You don't have to do a fast run or jog to get this feeling you can get in through other forms of exercise such as a quick walk around the block. Try and find a form of exercise that is something you personally will enjoy you will have a better chance of keeping it up if you enjoy it.

Relaxing Music:

Studies have shown that by listening to calming or soothing music it can help to lower blood pressure, anxiety and lower heart rate. You could arrange a selection on calming music that you can play perhaps while you are doing a yoga exercise that involves meditating. Listening to the calming music will help you to relax while you meditate. A popular choice of music for this is nature sounds such as birds chirping, waterfalls, ocean sounds etc.

Laughter is Good Medicine:

Who ever came up with the saying 'laughter is good medicine' could not have been more right. When a person engages in a good belly laugh this just doesn't reduce your mental stress but it lowers cortisol which is your body's stress hormone. So to help yourself lower your stress level try and laugh more; interact with those that put a smile on your face more or shows or movies that make you laugh. This is one of life's medicines that doesn't taste bad but makes you feel great!

Meditate:

You can help to lower your stress levels just by meditating for a few minutes a day. According to studies it is reported that meditation done on a daily basis may alter the brain's neural pathways, making you more able to withstand stress. All you have to do is sit up straight with your feet on the floor, close your eyes, choose a mantra such as "I feel at peace" and recite it out loud or silent. Let all other distracting thoughts pass by like clouds.

Slow Down:

By spending 5 minutes just focusing on the now and paying attention to your senses you will find that you feel less tense. An example would be if you are biting into a piece of food really focusing on chewing it slowly and savoring every bite. You will notice your senses becoming more in tune and alerting you more to your immediate surroundings.

Staying Connected:

It is very important that you stay connected with friends and loved ones sharing with them your thoughts and feelings. It is best if you can talk to someone face to face but if not then pick up the phone and call for some moral support. It is much healthier for you to talk about things that may be bothering you or causing you stress and worry. You can release some of your pent up anxiety by reaching out and talking with someone. Talking to a counselor is another option to get some advice on dealing with your stress.

Helping Others:

Research has shown that people who spend their money giving to charities or helping others feel happy about doing so. To help others doesn't mean you have to give a lot of time or money it could be a small action like giving a person a quarter so they can get a grocery cart. Just by smiling and saying hello to someone will make you feel better in knowing that there are good people in the world including yourself!

Chapter 4:
Finding Balance In Your Life

Combining Skills to Achieve Happiness:

You need to learn certain skills to know how to achieve happiness in place of worry and stress in your life. Research studies show that you do have some control over how happy you feel.

It is estimated that about 10% of your happiness is due to things in your life that are hard to change such as your income, your health, and your looks, 50% is decided by your genes and that leaves 40% up to you to decide this is the part that you can control. These skills can be difficult to acquire but as time goes by you will get better at using them as the saying goes 'practice makes perfect'.

Positive Relationships with Others:

Think about how connected you are with other people; do you tend to distance yourself from family and loved ones? How connected do you feel to others in general such as your neighbors, co-workers, if you don't feel close to others you should make an effort to try and become more social? Try and find others that have similar interests to your own that are positive in nature. Try and stay away from negative influences these will not help you to reach a less stressful lifestyle but will instead add to the stresses in your life.

Get Out of the House:

It is very healthy for you both mentally and physically to get out of the house and into the fresh outdoor air. Maybe you should think about joining a group such as a club, or take a class or check out the local religious groups in your area. These things can help you to get out of the house to meet new people and have some fun while doing so. Instead of sitting at home alone worrying about what isn't right with the world.

Well Rested:

Studies have shown that those who were well rested had more sense of well-being compared to those who were not well rested. So it is important to make sure that you get sufficient sleep so that you may function with all cylinders operating so to speak. If you are getting proper amounts of sleep, this will help to increase your happiness or contentment level.

Healthy Daily Habits:

Trying to change your bad habits is not going to be easy; but you can do things to make the transition a bit easier for yourself. Try and add positive things into your daily rituals such as adding an exercise routine. Stop eating heavy foods late at night and replace junk food snacks with healthier choices these are just a few examples. There are many healthy positive habits that you can choose from to add to your daily routine. Find some good habits that will be ones that you will be more than likely to continue for the long haul.

Stay Away from Alcohol:

If you are someone who suffers from depression you should try and avoid alcohol as it will just make your depression worse. You should try and keep away from alcohol as it will not help you to reach a true happy state in life; this you will find through making healthier choices and alcohol is not on that list. Some bad habits will be much harder to quit than others but the rewards you will reap will outweigh this tenfold.

Joining A Support Group:

A great way for you to get support while going through your journey towards seeking a happier way of life is a support group. If you are for example trying to lose weight but are finding it hard to do on your own then a good idea is to join a local weight watchers support group. This will be a great source to get encouragement to continue the battle to reach that healthier weight you want to get to. There is various support groups in most communities you just have to reach out and you will get the support you need to help guide you to a more stress free life.

Balancing Work and Play:

You must try and make an effort to set aside some down time or play time each and every day; don't rush through life working most of the time with no play this is not a healthy way to live. Many people spend far too much time doing work related things that they are missing out on the fun parts of life. You must remember that life is too short and you must not spend your precious time worrying and stressing about things. Instead you must make an effort to have some fun; try and laugh more and take things not too seriously all the time; learn to let your hair down and just enjoy all the positive and good things life has to offer for you!

Chapter 5:
Trying To Eat The Stress Away

Feel Better or Comfort Foods:

Many of us when we are feeling stressed or depressed we reach for the comfort foods that usually consist of junk food such as chips, chocolate, cake, cookies and ice-cream just to name a few. These foods belong to the group known as simple carbohydrates which are the bad fat group. These foods will give you a quick feel good feeling but before you know it the negative thoughts are back in full force. This can be caused by certain foods that can lower or raise your blood sugar levels or affect your body in other negative ways. Eating an unbalanced diet can have a great affect on your mood.

Choose a Healthy Snack:

Next time when you are craving that sweet snack instead of grabbing a cookie or piece of cake go for something that is healthy. Great healthy replacements are a piece of Melba toast and spread almond butter on it then top it with some slices of banana. This is a good replacement for cookies and cake. Starting this good eating habit will be life changing for you as it will lessen your negative moods as well as lessening the affect they have on you if they do occur.

Food the Modifier:

The brain is largely affected by the foods that we consume. Foods can be a great modifier when dealing with depression. By choosing meals and snacks that have a balance of several nutritional based parts this will strengthen your brain and body in ways that will help to boost your emotional health.

Magnesium Mood Booster:

Try and include magnesium-rich foods in your diet such as fish and sunflower seeds. Magnesium improves your mood by producing the brain chemical serotonin. Next time you are shopping try and add some of the following to your cart: pumpkin seeds, salmon, halibut, avocados, spinach, oats, peanuts, and almonds.

Omega- 3's Reduce Depression:

Scientific research has proven to show that the consumption of Omega-3's will reduce depression. Some foods high in Omega-3's include: tuna, Chia seeds, salmon, trout, sardines, and hemp. When you are choosing a type of fish try and pick one that is low in toxins such as mercury.

Nutritional Balance will Improve Emotional Balance:

By eating a well balanced diet you will improve your emotional balance. Why spend your time stressing over life when you can be enjoying it by eating a healthy balanced diet which will help to make you feel better both inside and out.

When your body is getting the nutrients it needs to function in a healthy way it will send signals out giving you that feel good feeling you are seeking. So why not start eating your way to a healthier happier version of you!

Chapter 6:
Remember To Be Grateful

You must try and focus on the good things in your life instead of looking and dwelling on the negative things. Don't spend your time mulling over past failures in your life but instead look at the positive events that occurred in your life. Remember the important thing is that no one in this world is perfect and we all make mistakes in life but learning from your mistakes is part of life's journey. Don't beat yourself up over a mistake you have made in life but instead move forward and learn from it.

Think of Others Who are in Need:

Take time in your life to stop and give thought to others in the world that is in dire need of help. Many people in the world suffer terribly not knowing where or if they will have a meal each and every day. They have no proper homes, no clean drinking water many die each and every day from ailments that they didn't have to die from. If they only had food and clean drinking water to sustain them like you have. These are people that would gladly trade places with you who have a home, food and clean drinking water but yet you are still unhappy.

Sometimes it takes looking at what others do not have to realize how much you do have and how blessed you are to have the life you have. It may not be your perfect idea of a life but that is up to you to make choices that will improve the quality of your life. At least you have the freedom and options to make choices for yourself many do not have the freedoms you have.

Stop Feeling Sorry for Yourself:

Instead of going on a self-pity trip perhaps you should instead try and focus on more positive things. When you feel yourself going into a depressive state where you think you are so hard done to stop and take a moment to think of all the people in the 3rd world countries that are dying of starvation each and every day while you sit feeling sorry for yourself.

Take this time and use it in a positive way such as making a donation to a charity either financial or by giving your time. You will feel much better than you would just lie around your home buried deep in a self-pity trip. You must get up and dust yourself off and begin taking actions in your life that will lead you to that happier life you seek but just remember to think about those who are less fortunate while doing so.

Show Compassion Towards Others:

Try and learn to have more compassion for those who may be homeless or in similar dire straits and think of ways that you can do your part to make the world a better place for all. Don't be afraid to go out into your community to find something that you may get involved with that is a good cause or group to join such as a religious based group.

Many religious groups help those in need; you could inquire what types of programs they may be involved in to help third world countries. Find a group or project that interests you in order to help others in need. You will get such a natural high from showing compassion and doing good things for those who are in great need of it.

Remember to Tell Your Loved Ones You Love Them:

A good habit to get into that will not only make your loved ones feel better in hearing it but it will also boost your mood is tell them you love them. Don't take your loved ones for granted and just presume that they know that you love them so you don't bother telling them. It is always nice to hear and reassuring when you hear a person say that they love you out loud. It helps to seal the bond with your loved ones keeping the relationships healthy by communicating clearly to others.

Don't cut yourself off from friends and family reach out to them for their support and you will get it. But you must be willing to let them know what is going on with you and try and talk about your feelings. Family counseling can be a good way to get some good advice on how to improve your relationships with loved ones. Try and be positive and give compliments to your loved ones not negative hurtful comments that can leave deep scars on a person's heart. If you have nothing good to say then don't say anything. If you think positive thoughts you should share them with others.

Giving Thanks Daily:

There is so much in life that you should be thankful for each and every day; try and give thanks on some level each and every day. Point out things that others do for you to make your life better each and every day and make sure you acknowledge these things and give thanks to those that give them to you. If you are a religious person remember to give thanks to your higher power for giving you the life you live today. But just remember the power to improve your life lies in your hands; you must be the one to take the steps towards the healthier happier life no one can take these steps for you.

Good luck in your journey to less worrying and more enjoying life to the fullest!

Chapter 7:
How Is Worrying Related To Living?

Like loose motions, pimples and flat tires, worrying has plagued everyone at some point of time or other. Worrying could be defined as the excessive brooding over things a person does even before the mentioned things could prove to be a problem. It involves over thinking about issues that in most cases, aren't even worth it. Everyone goes through daily life crisis and strives through the day to solve them. The process involved requires thinking and mental application of the best possible ways to sort things out.

Worrying, however, is not all negative. It is a necessary process to anticipate and get prepared for an unforeseeable problem. Imagine not stocking up extra tires at the back of your car before heading out for a picnic to an uneven terrain. Worry beforehand about the possible circumstances so you don't end up in trouble later. Worrying is an unconscious part of the various ways in which humans have learnt to survive. It is Darwin's way to make sure humans don't adopt a laid back attitude and be happy go lucky in life.

Worrying is a defense mechanism imbibed in humans to alert them of future issues. At times such issues are remote; while at other times these are imminent and deserve our special attention. It's the nature's way to put humans on their feet all the time. However, when practiced in abundance it can lead to health and life issues.

From being an alarm to being a stressful trait, worrying could change colors in minutes. It's that aspect of the human mind that keeps pushing for undivided attention to issues that don't deserve so much of mulling. Matters that could be solved by smart thinking and right decision making skills complicate themselves when they fall into the cockpit of worrying.

Despite the urgency, some issues could be tackled in shorter and better ways. The more you think about them, the more monstrous they appear. Such equations turn devastating for you in the end. It meets no end when you spend more than the required energy in things that could be solved in other ways and methods.

Worrying is therefore, an undesirable way to solving problems. Thinking when coupled with stress becomes worrying. It is not the over thinking that affects you; it's the consequences of such over thinking. You refuse to see any other way and choose to go the wrong way about solving problems. Your mind gets seized and shuts down any other and better alternatives that could have done the job quicker.

It is not only unhealthy for you but also time-consuming. You spend hours thinking over something so trivial that by the time you realize its non significance, it's already too late to start afresh and get done with it. Worrying complicates really simple things and doesn't allow you to think clearly. Minds should always be trained to avoid complex ways of tackling problems. He is a smart person who knows how to deal with issues in the quickest possible method.

Living hasn't been defined anywhere. No field of studies deals with as simple a concept as living. Despite that, it could be said to be an accumulation of activities that include more than mere animal existence of humans on earth. Life is a vast term with more than one meaning.

One aspect of it says it's about eating, sleeping and existing like a creature on earth. Another evolved version says living is about having rights. Yet another definition argues that living is more than just survival. It's about being able to maximize your happiness and minimize your pains. Benthamanian school of thought would define living to be something similar. The reduction of pain and heightening of pleasure could be summed up to be living.

In the contest of this eBook, living is going to be stretched as wide as possible. So what do you think living is? Is it working dully at your cubicle and earning money by the month? Or is it preparing dishes for your kids and seeing them off to school? It could be traveling from one place to another, just for the fun of it. Like it's been mentioned before, living cannot be bound by limits and definitions.

For one person living could have an entirely different meaning than the next person. Though it differs from person to person, there are some aspects of it that never change and everyone, regardless of where they are and how they are, are entitled to some of such basic benefits of living.

One of the most vital aspects of living is enjoyment. You have the right to enjoy while living. Human wants never cease. Be it in the form of a hobby or habit, wants never stop expressing themselves. We seek wants because we aim for enjoyment. Now is enjoyment possible at all the times? There are times when full enjoyment is not possible. More often than not, such times are created by the nuisance that we discussed at the start- worrying.

Worrying interferes with life. It diverts your attention and allots to it such irrelevant stuff that you cease to live. People are often afraid of failing and that causes them to worry to such an extent that they stop living at all. Or they end up living so cautiously that they might as well not have lived at all.

It's no life to be worrying about money and relationships. Life's more than about petty things. Sure, money is what keeps you going and relationships are necessary for one's romantic satisfaction but those things are not all life has got to offer. Look beyond such limiting concepts and discover an entire new definition of what you've been calling life so far. Explore new dimensions to life and set out to redefine living. Stop over thinking and start learning how to. You have got a limited time on this planet; why not make every minute count? Why is it mandatory that you spend every moment solving, and not living?

Chapter 8:
What Are The Primary Causes Of Worry?

Worrying causes you to shut down completely; so much so that you are no longer even available to alternatives that would have proved better than the current strategy you are planning to use. Worrying affects you in a variety of ways. This chapter deals with such effects and their consequences in detail.

Insecurity

Insecurity is both, a cause and a result of worry. The word 'insecurity' maybe defined as that feeling of human mind which propels it to feel threatened in one way or another. Such a threatening could be from a friend or a colleague. Insecurity either leads to worries or worries themselves create insecurities.

It is perfectly normal to feel insecure in today's life. Life has turned into a rat race and every competing rat feels insecure about the next in line. Rats fight among themselves while running towards the elusive and non existing end. They do not realize there is none.

There must have been instances where you felt insecure. The pressure the corporate world has to offer to its employees makes it hard for anyone to escape the evil of insecurity. Let me give you an example of how insecurity plays its role:

Fred and Harvey are co-workers at a top corporate firm. Fred is a senior while Harvey is a clerk but both are good friends who entered the office around the same year. So far so good! One day, the top boss appoints a very easy task to Harvey and is promised a promotion upon its completion. Such a promotion would escalate Harvey's position to almost the same level as Fred. Fred complains to the boss about such an opportunity not being presented to him. The boss calls him out on this complaint in a meeting which was attended by Harvey too.

Two things happened. First, Fred lost whatever goodwill he had accumulated in the eyes of his boss. And second, he also lost the trust of his friend Harvey who now knows that Fred is insecure about him.

Insecurity is good at times though. It is not always a bad thing. By being insecure, you derive the required zeal to win and keep competing. But there comes a time when it exceeds the optimum level and turns adverse. Insecurity when exercised in abundance leads to bad situations like the one discussed above. It is to be sparingly acted upon, and if possible, completely avoided.

Jealousy

The difference between insecurity and jealously is that insecurity involves a threat to one's own interests while jealously requires a person to compare oneself with others. Both the traits however, end up involving comparison and relativity with regards to someone else.

Jealousy could be described as the feeling of wishing for something to be brought within your personal interest at the cost of someone else's rights which are currently being used with regards to the thing in question.

There however, is an obvious difference between jealousy and envy. Enviousness is the term referring to a person's positive wishing while jealousy is more on the negative side of one's mind. When one is envious regarding a thing, one doesn't wish for that thing to be snatched away from the current possessor or user.

Enviousness usually is used in situations where the envious person is drawing inspiration from a brilliant work. Say, if I see a beautiful painting, I'd say I'm envious of the painter who possesses such an amazing skill to paint. In the same situation, if I were a painter myself, I'd have been probably jealous and not envious, unless I am too principled a man.

Jealousy is an obvious cause for worry. It makes you burn to ashes while wishing for someone else to suffer the same. Jealousy propels you to even act on the feeling and cause harm to others, just for the sole intention to separate them from the thing you are wishing for, or somehow cease the enjoyment of your targeted thing by its owner or user. It is not possible to right away eliminate jealousy; more so if you are in a workplace.

People get rewards for their works. If you work hard and smart enough, so will you. Being jealous of someone from work is a major reason for corporate pressure. It is not always possible to be at your best in order to keep impressing your corporate daddies. Sometimes, you have to be satisfied with the mundane. Pull out of the race once in a while to hang your boots and relax.

Completely shutting you down would backfire though. Keep a lookout for competition and prospective chances of promotion and reward gaining. But whenever someone else receives the same, try to be nice instead of jealous. You can't get everything you want. If you did, everyone would have everything on earth and there would be no worries in the first place.

Competitions

Life itself is a big competition. But it's filled with tiny and unimportant competitions that when taken together decide whether you have won the big race or not.

You face competition in every walk of your life. Be it your neighborhood club or your office, competition keeps popping its head out in some form or other. Competition is healthy as long as it is limited to fun and participation.

The moment it turns into a struggle, trouble calls. Unhealthy and excessive competitive environments like corporate offices and a posh neighborhood could prove adverse for you. While competition is good to decide who the best is, for those who lose it or are in a habit of losing, there remains no enjoyment in competing and they end up worrying about it.

Remember the last time you visited Mrs. Next Door and felt envious of the newly bought Japanese vase kept proudly on their centre table? Or gave your fellow worker a cold stare when he completed the task allotted to you in less than the time you took to do it?

Competition exists everywhere. All you got to do is take a look around and you will find competition from the cab stand to the corporate world. Sometimes, people are so consumed by competitions that they start taking it as seriously as would affect their normal functioning; mental and physical. They are immersed in the possibility of winning and are ready to think over plans and plots to do so. Having invested so much of their physical, mental and economic resources into competitions, people completely ignore the negative effects competitions have on them.

Stress and strain

No one's aloof from daily life stress. Right from the moment your electric bill shoots up more than the usual digit to when your kids' school reports fly in the door, you experience stress and strain in numerous forms and sizes.

Stress has become so much of an ingrained part of our lives that one moment without it raises suspicion. Its absence is unimaginable since in an ideal set up of today's life; stress has to play a part somewhere. When it goes missing, funnily, people find something amiss. Peace and tranquility have been reduced to mere dictionary words that are no longer in practical usage; except whilst mentioning their absence.

Stress could be defined as the mental agony one goes through because of excessive pressure with regards to someone, something or some place. Stress is harmful not only for you but also for those who are close to you. It is not a nice experience to live in a household where its members are stressed and unhappy. Cold porridge poured by a smiling mother is better than a luxurious lunch course served by a frowning one.

Stress cannot be considered a cause for worry but rather one would address stress to be an extreme and heightened form of worrying. Worrying could invade your mind any time. But stress requires some real problematic issues that have been eating you up since long. It takes more than a few thoughts to build up stress. A mere reflection constitutes a worry while an accumulation of such reflection coupled with negative thinking leads to stress.

Priorities

Everyone has a mental arrangement of priorities that get ticked one by one as you travel through the day. Priorities are importance oriented things that one has in mind. Not everything is important to you. You do not allot the same relevance to every person, thing, event and place that comes across you.

Priorities can cause worry in three ways. One, when priorities aren't met. Second, when they swap places causing a panic attack. And third, when they are so ambitious that you realize they can't be met.

Let's talk about these three ways in which priorities can cause worry in detail.

The first way is when priorities aren't met. We all have such things in our lives that we assign relevance to, yes? These things could be someone, something or some event. When we have put so much of our investment in achieving or using something, we naturally expect to receive it. When we don't, our priorities tumble down the hole and we end up worrying about the lost chances.

The second way in which priorities can affect us, causing us to over think is when they swap places. We cannot assign the same priority status to two different things. Let me help you with an illustration here.

Susan is a happily married woman who balances her job and household life quite well. She happens to be a talented designer and a dutiful wife. Off late, she's been assigned a pile of work at her office due to which she's been coming late to home, often post dinner. Such a behavioral change has aroused doubts in her husband's mind as to Susan's character. He's insecure about her spending too little time with him and their kids. When he conveys this feeling to Susan, her world breaks down and she starts worrying what went wrong.

It was only later that she realizes that her priorities have been unintentionally swapped. Her work had taken over her role as a wife and there was nothing she could do to prevent it. Both the roles, worker and wife, were initially assigned the same priority but now, one has gone ahead in the race and reached a lead.

Such situations that reveal a change in priorities have a tendency to push someone spiraling into depths of worrying.

The final and most devastating cause of worry under this heading is the most notorious of all. Imagine loving someone thinking they harbor similar feelings towards you. You get into a relationship with them and everything is rosy for a while until you realize the other person has fallen out and is now, bored of your company.

What used to be your top priority was nothing but an illusion. Some priorities need a reply. They need to be reacted upon or responded to. It's mostly in case of relationships that we witness the third way in which worry is injected in human minds. It's caused not because of a change in priorities but the realization of its non-existence from the beginning.

Expectations

An expectation is a wishful thought that assumes other people to perform, behave, act or speak in a certain manner. Expectation could be best summed up as that part of the mind that wants something in return from people.

We all have expectations; tiny, big, mundane, brilliant, unfulfilled, met, unmet; the sorts are too many to be categorized. It's natural to expect. It is also natural to go into a seizure mode when they are not fulfilled. But what is not natural is that you have unreasonable ones.

Having expectations is good; having impossible ones is not. It's always good to keep your feet grounded and see the practical picture before diving to create unreasonable expectations. It's not bad to dream, but to make castles in the air? No.

Relationships, academics, office, if expectations were able to appear in the form of tiny flags over people's heads, the world would have been turned into a race course. When our expectations aren't met we worry. When our expectations are crushed after being met, we worry. When our expectations reveal themselves to be an unreal one, we worry. Majority of our worry derives its inspiration from expectations not turning real.

Survival

Survival is the struggle for existence faced by all men equally. It is the race which is run by everyone in order to keep living. Survival issues exist in the form of thinking about money, home, kids and livelihood.

Right from the day Darwin gave his theory of survival; of how the fittest come out winners in a jungle, it has been accepted as a norm that humans are not excluded from it. It is a law of nature that in order to exist, one has to fulfill some basic needs. Survival of the fittest is only one aspect of the Darwin theory; those who run the race include fit people and not everyone is the fittest. To ensure survival in today's world, the mentioned essentials like money, home and livelihood are among the top priorities of anyone willing to run the race.

Some people achieve these basic amenities with ease and talent. On the other hand, for others, it becomes a continuous struggle. The number of unemployed people in the world is alarming; so is the figure of underfed and homeless people. Such issues present themselves as huge challenges to survival and eventually turn into primary causes of worry.

Chapter 9:
How To Minimize Or Eliminate Worry From Your Life?

It is quite simple to tackle worry. Let me walk you through a series of ways in which you can minimize worries and even uproot them from your life.

You can't be worry-free overnight. Those who are in a constant state of worrying, it becomes difficult to switch out from it and start living a normal life. Worry is so deeply imbibed in our lives that a sudden uprooting is not possible and the treatment prescribed requires cleverness, patience and hard work.

Food

What problem on earth can't be cured by food? Be it a bad mood or a terminal disease, it all comes down to food when the treatment stage is entered into. It has been observed that food keeps you balanced and running. Often, worrying people skip their meals in order to spend time and energy whining over petty matters. This further leads to health degradation and worrying gets pronounced even more disastrously than before.

Prepare a diet plan of you own. Include the following items in it without a fail: Green leafy vegetables, ripe fruits, sprouts, meat (optional), juice, red beef, pork, eggs, milk and assorted beans. Besides the mentioned food items, you can also go for your favorite munchies but make sure they are not stale or too fatty.

Stick to your dietary chart, regardless of what you weigh. A planned diet often helps one take his mind off things that cause distractions leading to worries. When you have a fixed diet, you will make sure it is religiously followed so as to not upset your health. By sticking to the plan sincerely, you leave little room for worry to creep in.

Planning

Always make plans. Even if it's for a faraway event that is yet to knock at your attention's door, be prepared for it in advance. Here are some of the ways in which you can lead a planned lifestyle:

Maintain a daily journal that should contain all your important appointments, dates, timings and places of shenanigans you have to attend, manage or take care of. That way, you won't end up missing out or neglecting any of them. It even helps you create a mental priority list of sorts wherein those works very important to you would assume top positions and those that can suffer delay would assume the low positions.

In addition to a daily journal, get into the habit of keeping a monthly journal which would contain less regular affairs like dentist visits, parents meetings at school, bills to be paid for electricity, water and cable and other such stuff that don't need so constant an attention.

Never allot an appointment such a time as it would make it difficult for you to attend it. It serves no purpose when you don't attend an appointment on time since neither party stands to gain from it. Keep spaces for travel and eating between two appointments so as to not fall into the habit of rushing.

Inculcate the habit of scrapbooking in your kids. Scrapbooking is a fun way to not only keep track of what's happening in your life but also to slowly but surely usher in a habit of organization.

Keep at least one day in the weekend free. This time has to be allotted for family activities like going out for movies, picnic or a simple excursion to the local museum. Do not let your kids felt ignored while you are caught up in your busy life. A day a week may not be sufficient for you to really get involved with the kids. Keep a track of their assignments from time to time and make sure you ensure their overall development by asking them to join extracurricular activities.

Planning is an art which when learnt could reap huge benefits. It is planning alone that could keep your life in order. The less chaotic your life is, the more worry-free it remains. Order is important for any human to find peace within himself. If you remain a disoriented and unorganized person, it affects not just you but also your family.

Say, you are a housewife who is responsible for dinner preparation in your home. Now, if you end up neglecting this responsibility of yours due to social kitty parties in your neighborhood, it could lead to kids falling asleep without their supper and developing a bad habit of not gaining the required nutrition for an average child to grow. It could even result in disruption of family peace which in turn could assume the shape of a major worry.

Socialization

With the fast shrinking of world due to fast and better technology, people are falling out of the habit of real life socializing. What used to describe one's personality in older times has become a neglected part of our lives. Some decades ago, the more one socialized, the better the chances of him being perceived a balanced person. Today, socialization has reduced to such extent that it's almost considered a dying form of getting to know people.

Social networking sites like Facebook and twitter have taken over and people's worries and problems are shared online, among internet friends. If you feel bad about being slapped a pay cut due to low productivity as a worker, you are more likely to go online and make a status than facing and solving the issue by contacting your boss.

Socializing in real life has a variety of benefits for those wallowing in a corner with a truckload of worries to look after.

When you socialize you meet people who might be undergoing similar issues as you, or even larger and worse ones. Upon coming to learn of them, you connect to them and feel relieved. Socializing has a calming effect on people as it prevents them from feeling alone.

Sharing is caring. We are all familiar with this old proverb which still holds true. When you meet people in real life and share your problems, you receive not only sympathy but also practical solutions to such problems. They no longer remain your issues as there's someone else who shares the load of it with you.

Imagine a worry to be the number 16. When you tell it to the first person, he takes away eight and you are left with eight. When you tell it to the second person, you are left with four, then two and then subsequently one. This is how worry-sharing works. The more you share, the lesser it keeps becoming.

Escape

Escape has long been used as a word used to describe people who aren't brave. Its width and scope however, is broader than that. Escape is a way which one chooses when things don't go one's way.

It is okay to choose an escape to get away from things troubling you. Any place or thing could be chosen as an escape. Even a person could be an escape.

Want to find your escape? Look for things that distract your mind from things that tense you. It could be a Harry Potter novel, or a peaceful park. It could even be your best friend who keeps talking about hobbits. Escaping away is not a sin; it's not an act of cowardice. On the other hand, it is refusing to deal with things that damage you. It is placing a firm foot down and claiming your right to not face a negative thing for either some time, or ever.

When you escape a worry, you don't run from it. You simply ignore it. Now, ignoring a worry isn't solving it. But worrying won't either. Why not allow yourself some quiet which could potentially heal you back to your normal state of mind and then you could take on the problem with a fresh and better perspective? Escaping is one the best ways to tackle issues. You haven't completely run from it; you have only delayed its appointment till the time you are fully ready to tackle it.

Positivity

Why not try a little dose of positivity in your life? Maybe you are full of so many worries because you are in a negative environment that doesn't even allow positive thoughts to surround you? Worrying is a state of mind and not being.

Despite that being true, there are physical entities that could affect the way in which you deal with worries.

Suppose you are sitting in your cubicle when your boss emails you about a possible demotion unless you submit the required work within a week. Now, if there are flowers on your table, a picture of your family framed in beautiful putty and a freshly laid cloth, you are more likely to start working on the work and finish it within a week than when you are working in a dull environment.

It is quite easy to instill positivity around yourself. All you have to do is take care of some simple things.

Start everyday with something fresh. A fruit, a flower, your kid's giggle, or glasses of fresh orange juice- take your pick. It's the start of the day that dictates how the rest of the day is going to unfurl as.

Mingle with everyone at your workplace and greet them with a smile. Make sure your office environment not only remains friendly but also genuine. Get rid of those people who inspire negative thoughts in your mind and make friends with those that you consider good mates to socialize with.

Go out drinking once in a while with your romantic partner or friends. Reserve the Saturday of every week to go out on such fun activities since Sunday would most likely b spent on bed, having woken up from a nice hangover. You could allot Sunday for family time fun by preparing a nice lunch and going out fishing together.

Prevent yourself from falling into the bad habits of back bitching and gossiping. Such things are considered not only bad traits but also the surest way to lead to worry. Do not form an opinion on someone just from a first impression as they can often be misleading. Get to know the person well before judging. Mind your tongue whilst speaking. It's the tongue that does most of the damage. Choose words wisely and compliment people on their looks, achievements and for simply existing in your life.

Positivity is a habit. It changes your perception of the world and your personal opinion about a lot of things. A positive person is more likely to stay worry free than a negative person.

Learn to say no

A lot of people get pushed into a plethora of worries only because they aren't versed with the art of saying no. 'No' is a two lettered word that requires the mightiest of courage to say it. Often people invite worries because they couldn't say no at the right time.

Learning to say no is an art all of you should master. Not everything in the world deserves your attention or indulgence. There are things that interest you and there are others that don't. The first step to say no is categorizing these two kinds of things. You may want to have a bottle of beer on your weekend but when you go there in a group you are forced to go for whiskey only because the entire group is having it. Such situations call for a polite no, followed by opting for your choice of drink.

Let's take another illustration.

A guy has been pursuing you romantically since a month. A time comes when harangued by his attempts and advances; you give in and accept to be in a relationship with him. After a week of this, you come to realize that not only is he not your type, but he's also cheating on you. You get into depression and start worrying about your relationship.

This illustration is different from the previous one in the sense that in the former you had to avoid a bad situation with politeness while the latter required putting a firm foot down and refusing to stand back. The urgency to say no was more in the latest illustration.

The intensity with which a no has to be pronounced also matters. It reflects on how your mental set up at the time of saying no. Regardless, it doesn't matter what state of mind you are in; if you are saying a no, it should mean so. Not being able to say it at the proper time, to the right person may prove itself a catalyst for worries.

Develop hobbies

There are always such times during the day when you do nothing; times of leisure, if you will. Fill these empty gaps with activities you would like to get into. Make sure there is no such time of the day that isn't occupied by anything interesting.

Developing hobbies not only further your passion towards certain habits, but also keeps your mind off trivial matters. Your attention has a fixed quota. Utilize this to the fullest capacity by spending it on something creative and fun rather than something petty. What is even better is the possibility that this hobby may add value to your overall personal development.

Professional life v. Personal life

If you happen to be one of those corporate honchos who find it difficult to find time for their families, change it. Make sure that your personal life isn't confined to arriving just time for dinners and leaving for office even before your kids wake up. Do not bring home pile of work from the office. Do not fall into the habit of receiving office calls during morning breakfasts. If it's feasible, drop your kids off at their school on your way to office.

Surprise your family by suddenly turning up from work to take them dining out. Very rare things can replace such pleasant surprises. This will not only please the kids, but also reassure your better half about your concern for the family. Such attempts help you keep worries out of your marital life.

A good balance must be struck between your professional and personal life. Either shouldn't be allowed to overlap with the other. Most divorce cases in the United States in the last five years have happened because of the very reason that people's professional lives and personal lives intermingled.

Yoga

Yoga is an accumulation of body exercises that directly affect your state of mind. Learn yoga from a yoga instructor or check YouTube for practically free yoga sessions that are uploaded by Indian swamis and practitioners.

Yoga exercises help a person remove unwanted worries by clearing the pathway of his thinking process. Increased oxygen supply to the brain ensures smooth functioning of your analytical process. There are asanas (Sanskrit for postures) that increase your memory power and help you focus your concentration only on things that matter to you.

Stay healthy, if not fit

Your body has a say in how your mind functions. Without a healthy body, your mind is, if it's not now, soon to become defunct. It is said that to ensure a person's insanity, it is important that he first pays attention to his health. This shows how vital it is to stay healthy.

It is not necessary that you have a well toned body after hitting six months of gym. To address worries, you first need to become physically fit. Your mind must be capable enough to comprehend the difference between irrelevant and relevant matters. This comprehension is the first step towards worry elimination. Once you have the knowledge of what is important and what is not, you are half equipped to tackle worries.

Eat a healthy diet throughout the year. Hit a gym if you want to, but it's not mandatory. Take care of obesity as it may lead to mental disorders later in your life. Keep clear of medications unless they are very important to be taken.

Another aspect of health maintenance is checking or preventing drug use. Alcohol isn't a drug per se but its effects are no lesser than one. Wine is good for health but only when consumed on occasional circumstances and small quantities. Do not fall into a habit of smoking as it may lead to serious consequences. Not only that, it may also push you further into the world of addiction which is a breeding ground of worries.

Do not neglect your sleep and food cycles. Sleep and rise early. Make sure you sleep soon after your dinner. Rising early has its own benefits. It's said that the early morning sun is the best source of vitamin D. The fresh air out in the local park could just prove to be a good trigger for the day. It's always wise to start your day afresh and a jog in the sun could provide you exactly that.

Coming to food cycles, never miss the most the three most important meals of the day – breakfast, lunch and dinner. Regardless of how busy your life is, skipping these three supreme meals of the day will surely going to have a bad effect on your overall health. In addition to these three, take time out for little snacks in between. Such snacks ensure food's entry into your system thereby revitalizing you with the necessary energy supplements.

Prevention is always better than cure. Why not lead a healthy life from the start and avoid worries rather than neglect your health and facing issues later? A physically sound body ensures a mentally fit mind. Your mind is the source of all worries. Keep it up and running and it will automatically combat your worries for you.

Chapter 10:
How To Prevent Worries From Aggravating

A worry is a very small term used for an issue. An issue arises when a worry is aggravated to extreme limits and bounds. A worry turns into an issue when it is thought upon to such extent that its threat multiplies and it turns into more dangerous forms than when it was a mere worry.

The previous chapter focused on ways to prevent worry. This chapter however, will deal with ways to cure worries; a stage which is reached after worries have already started invading your mental faculties.

First stage: Identification

How do you recognize something's been worrying you? The answer is simple. If something is occupying too much of your mental energy and isn't getting solved after many attempts of trying hard, it's a worry.

It is very important to spot a worry when it's in its initial stages; otherwise it may take a monstrous form and present itself to you as a looming hurdle to a normal life.

Second stage: Treatment

There are two ways to treat a worry, once it has been identified. You could either cure it or you could abandon it because of how least valuable it is to you.

A worry can prove to be disastrous if not addressed. This is when you take up arms and cure it. However, there a lot of worries which don't need the tiniest of your attention. Learn to ignore such worries and move forward in life.

Third stage: Alienation

Now that the worry has either been abandoned or cured, ensure your complete isolation from the worry. It often happens that we tend to return to our worries. Worries are to be abandoned never to be gotten back to. If you have successfully eradicated a worry, it is gone from your life forever, never to return, unless you want it to. Prevent yourself from over thinking about it especially after you have closed the lid on it.

Fourth stage: Unconscious imbibing of the three stages

Now, it is not expected of you that you remember all the three stages as per the given directions. But with constant practice and regular usage, you will learn to reproduce these stages without a hiccup or flaw. Being able to unconsciously heal yourself through a worry is an art you need to master in order to be well armed to battle everyday worries.

Over thinking kills the game. Do not brood over anything that doesn't deserve it. Learn to categorize your priorities. However if something is even remotely relevant, do not ignore its red alert signal. Do not get confused between a worry and something that needs urgent attendance. You'd do better to rather utilize this time to pursue hobbies and paying attention to matters that are in fact, relevant to you.

Resist going into a panic mode. Worrying is like drowning. The more you struggle by flapping your limbs, the farther down you sink. It's the panic stage that helps aggravation of worries the most. Keep as calm as is humanly possible. Seek psychiatric assistance and make sure you end up attending all the prescribed sessions. Be frank in such sessions and do not hesitate to open up even if it requires delving into personal details and dirty history.

Aggravation of worries can be prevented by either curing them or finding ways to get rid of them. Now it's not always possible to find a cure. Such circumstances call for actions along the lines of "Ignorance is Bliss". Take precautions against too much of ignorance as such a behavior may result into neglect of important matters.

Chapter 11:
How Would Stopping Worrying Help You With Start Living?

Some wise man has rightfully said "Don't worry be happy". So is there any point in worrying? Worrying is an emotion which can interfere with your normal state of mind at any point of time.

As per psychology, Worry has been described as the response to a challenge faced by a person with the inadequate skills to face the same. Worrying can be for both short lived and long lived moments. For eg: A student, who has to appear for an exam, worries for a short span of time (days or weeks) till the exam is over whereas in another case couples start worrying from the very moment they come to know that the female partner is pregnant up till the day of delivery that is scheduled to take place after nine months.

Everything has its own merits and demerits and worrying is no exception to it. Worrying has both negative and positive effects for eg: Over-worrying can give a person high anxiety levels which may lead to increased blood pressure and this will ultimately have a negative ulterior effect on your mental and physical health.

Moreover, over-worrying can seriously interfere with your sleep cycles leading you to suffer with insomnia at a later point of time. Moderate worrying allows a person to take precautions and other safety measures beforehand such as applying for different kinds of insurance or avoiding binge food and drinking habits.

It is a matter of common knowledge that there are four phases of life which are

i) Baby phase

ii) ii) Adolescent phase

iii) iii) Youth phase

iv) iv) Old phase

There are absolutely Zero levels of worrying during the first phase. Levels of worrying tend to rise up during your adolescent phase which basically is the student phase. The basic worry during this phase comes from exam and peer pressures.

During the third phase, one may experience peak levels of worry as during this phase people might be concerned about various things for eg: fulfilling the basic need of livelihood, one might be playing the role of a mother or father, who is concerned about the wellness of their progeny, societal pressure etc. During your last phase, as a person grows older, levels of worrying tend to diminish day by day, but this again is subject to exceptions.

Reports and surveys show that females tend to worry more as compared to men. One big reason for such conclusion might be women's general attribute of being more emotional by nature as compared to the nature of a man.

A child living at a different place may at random moments get calls from his/her mother and these calls are made in order to ascertain the wellness of a child. Such instances illustrate how the female part of the biodiversity is more inclined to worrying as opposed to the male part.

One of the main causes of worrying is people being concerned about their loved ones. It is pretty obvious that one will not worry about strangers but his relatives, friends, colleagues, kith and keens generally remain on top of his list. Another reason of worrying can be that a person is concerned with his or her image. Another big factor which adds up to worrying is the need for earning bread and shelter for yourself and your family.

People go haywire by going from one place to another place, talking to strangers, dealing with them and their egos, practicing the art of sycophancy just to ensure their livelihood. Another cause of worrying may arise from one's wish to prove their ability in front of the world. Starting from sportspersons, celebrities, lawyers, doctors, pedagogues and so on, everyone just wants themselves to be at the top.

Worrying is a behavior which is not just the attribute of human beings. Animals also worry, especially the female species that care about their little ones. Birds have a tendency to first hunt for the food and then they carry the same in their mouths up to their nests for the purpose of feeding their babies. One may have experienced the intimidation from a bitch, when he or she was busy playing with her puppies.

Levels of worrying may depend upon person to person. Some people may start worrying about happenings of some insubstantial events and some people are too lazy and ignorant to even pay heed on life changing situations.

It is indeed true that any other person cannot understand completely the reasons of worrying which the concerned person might have because of the very reason that every person is unique and this uniqueness is reflected on their different perceptions regarding worrying in different situations of lives.

There are many ways to tackle worry. Sharing one's problems with their family members can be a good way to start with. Socialization with people can also be fruitful because it has been scientifically proved that when a person shares his or her problems with their close buddies, he is relieved off his pressure.

Another key to relieve oneself from worrying is to engage oneself daily with the act of meditation. It is believed that the best time for meditation is early in the morning during which one can expect to inhale more levels of fresh oxygen. This ancient art of living is very effective in giving you a kick-start for the day which is in a way fruitful for your pursuit to fight with the world, with regards to your day to day activities.

Another good way to deal with worrying is to take rest at proper intervals and duly sleep time to time. It is always advised to maintain a daily routine so that things don't get mixed up leading to complexity in one's life. After conducting a study, it has come into light that early risers face less stress or fatigue levels at the end of the day as compared to any other person who is nonchalant about his or her sleep-cycles.

Another step in lowering down one's level of worrying is to find the right partner, with whom one can share his grieves and miseries provided that the partner is compatible with one's persona. In a love relationship, a person is relieved off the worrying when his or her companion consorts the person with their presence and intimacies. A warm hug or a kiss in a way is very effective.

Some research works have also shown that keeping pets such as dogs or cats can also decrease levels of worrying. Just imagine a situation where you have to go home after dealing with the cruel world and upon arriving at your place all exhausted, a little furry tongue wagging is waiting for you to greet you and starts licking you on your arrival showing its unconditional love and affection for you.

Apart from all these, one of the most common ways of releasing the pressure of worrying is to engage oneself into intoxication. It's a general trend that people smoke and drink. These may be temporary, but these may fit into the phrase of "need of the hour", provided when there is too much of worrying. However, it is always to be kept in mind that too much of intoxication may lead to addiction which may act as a catalyst for already existing worries.

Living has been hailed as more than just existence. Worrying is a leech that sucks one's life dry. It is vital to one's living that worrying be kept at bay and life be given the front of the line.

Conclusion

Thank you again for downloading this book!

I hope this book was able to help you to start living your life as you should.

The next step is to apply what you've learned on a daily basis.

Finally, if you enjoyed this book, please take the time to share your thoughts and post a review on Amazon. It'd be greatly appreciated!

Thank you and good luck!

Printed in Great Britain
by Amazon